KETO FLAVORS COOKBOOK

Low Carb Homemade Sauces, Rubs, Marinades, Butters & More

Infuse Fresh Flavors into Your
Everyday Keto Cuisine

INTRODUCTION

Keto recipes do not have to be just another flavorless meal. Keto food should not be about how many grams of fat and net carbs you are consuming, it should be about the taste and flavors, you should *enjoy* every meal. Adding any of the sauces, infused oils, dips or any recipe from this book to your meal will bring it alive with flavor and even provide a fiery kick (if that is what you like). All safe in the knowledge you can still maintain your low carbohydrate or keto diet.

Here's what makes each of these keto sauces great:

- No added sugar
- No artificial ingredients
- Use of whole and natural ingredients
- Low in carbs
- Bursting with flavor
- Easy to make

On the following contents page, each recipe has several labels for your ease of use.

Dietary labels

GF – The recipe is gluten free

DF – The recipe is dairy free

V – The recipe is vegetarian

The recipes goes well with:

Meat – a meat based dish

Fish – a fish based dish

Vegetarian – a vegetarian based dish

TABLE OF CONTENTS

Introduction 2

Must-have Keto Sauce Ingredients 11

How to Store Your Keto Sauces Like a Pro 12

How This Book Works 13

Final words 16

Sauces 17

Quick and Easy Pesto (GF, V) (Meat or Vegetarian) 18

Creamy Garlic Cheddar Sauce (GF) (Meat or Vegetarian) 19

Marinara Sauce (GF, V) (Vegetarian, Meat, Fish) 20

"Penne" Vodka Sauce (GF) (Meat, Vegetarian, Fish) 21

Sweet Butter Sauce (GF) (Meat) 22

Alfredo Parmesan Sauce (GF) (Meat) 23

Almond Butter Sauté Sauce (DF, GF) (Meat, Vegetarian) 24

Dill Hollandaise Sauce (GF) (Meat, Vegetarian) 25

Sour Cream and Onion Sauce (GF) (Meat) 26

Creamy Vegetable Sauce (GF) (Vegetarian) 27

Hot Sauces

............28

Traditional Hot Sauce (DF, GF) (Meat, Vegetarian)..................29

Creamy Jalapeño Hot Sauce (GF) (Meat) 30

Curry Hot Pepper Sauce (DF, GF) (Meat, Vegetarian)............31

Chili Paste (DF, GF) (Meat)..32

Spicy Red and Yellow Pepper Sauce (DF, GF) (Meat, Vegetarian) 33

Spicy Tomato Sauce (DF, GF) (Meat, Vegetarian) 34

Dressings

............35

Blue Cheese Dressing (GF) (Meat, Vegetarian)......................36

Ranch Dressing (GF) (Meat, Vegetarian)............................37

Caesar Dressing (GF) (Meat, Vegetarian)...........................38

Balsamic Vinaigrette (DF, GF) (Meat, Vegetarian)..................39

Italian Olive Oil Dressing (DF, GF) (Meat, Vegetarian, Fish) 40

Basil Avocado Dressing (GF) (Meat, Vegetarian)....................41

Lemon Honey Mustard Dressing (DF, GF) (Meat, Vegetarian, Fish)....42

Parsley Lemon Dressing (DF, GF) (Meat, Vegetarian, Fish) 43

Dips

............44

Spicy Mustard Dipping Sauce (GF) (Meat, Vegetarian) 45

Clove and Basil Mustard Sauce (GF) (Meat, Vegetarian) 46

Baked Bacon and Garlic Dip (GF) (Meat)...........................47

Caramelized Onion Cream Cheese Dip (GF) (Meat) 48

Spicy Chili Pepper Dip (GF) (Meat)...............................49

Creamy Herb Dip (GF) (Meat, Vegetarian)...50

Crushed Red Pepper and Garlic Dip (DF, GF) (Meat)....................................51

Cranberry Cottage Cheese Dip (GF) (Vegetarian)......................................52

Sour Cream and Cucumber Dip (GF) (Vegetarian).....................................53

Guacamole (DF, GF) (Meat, Vegetarian)...54

Spicy Guacamole (DF, GF) (Meat, Vegetarian)..55

Condiments

Condiments...56

Mayonnaise (DF, GF) (Meat, Vegetarian)...57

Chipotle Mayonnaise (DF, GF) (Meat, Vegetarian)....................................58

Ketchup (DF, GF) (Meat, Vegetarian)..59

Mustard (DF, GF) (Meat, Vegetarian)..60

BBQ Sauce (DF, GF) (Meat, Vegetarian)...61

Marinades

Marinades...62

Grilled Chicken Marinade (DF, GF) (Meat)..63

Caribbean Chicken Marinade (DF, GF) (Meat)...64

Spicy Chicken Marinade (DF, GF) (Meat)..65

Italian Marinade (DF, GF) (Meat, Vegetarian)...66

Jerk Chicken or Fish Marinade (DF, GF) (Meat, Fish)................................67

Mediterranean Marinade (DF, GF) (Meat, Fish)..68

Lemon and Herb Marinade (DF, GF) (Meat, Fish).....................................69

Classic Steak Marinade (DF, GF) (Meat)...70

Balsamic and Mustard Steak Marinade (DF, GF) (Meat)............................71

Teriyaki Marinade (DF, GF) (Meat)..72

Butter Marinades

Butter Marinades 73

Dill and Butter Marinade (GF) (Meat, Fish)......................................74

Garlic and Chive Marinade (GF) (Meat)..75

Herbed Butter Marinade (GF) (Meat, Fish)......................................76

Steak Butter Marinade (GF) (Meat)..77

Olive Oil and Butter Shrimp Marinade (GF) (Fish).........................78

Seasonings and Rubs

Seasonings and Rubs 79

Classic Italian Seasoning (DF, GF) (Meat, Fish, Vegetarian)...........80

Taco Seasoning (DF, GF) (Meat)...81

Fajita Seasoning (DF, GF) (Meat)..82

Seasoned Salt Rub (DF, GF) (Meat, Fish)..83

Ranch Seasoning (DF, GF) (Meat)...84

Curry Powder (DF, GF) (Meat, Vegetarian)......................................85

Chili Powder (DF, GF) (Meat)...86

Adobo Seasoning (DF, GF) (Meat)...87

Blackened Seasoning (DF, GF) (Meat, Fish)......................................88

Pumpkin Spice Seasoning (DF, GF) (Vegetarian)............................89

Glazes and Infused Oils

Glazes and Infused Oils 90

Garlic and Thyme Oil (DF, GF) (Meat, Fish, Vegetarian) 91

Garlic and Rosemary Oil (DF, GF) (Meat, Fish, Vegetarian)..........92

Ginger Chicken Glaze (DF, GF) (Meat)...93

Balsamic Steak Glaze (DF, GF) (Meat)...94

Butter Steak Glaze (GF) (Meat)...95

Dessert Sauces 96

Caramel Sauce (GF)..97

Hot Fudge Sauce (GF) 98

Apple Cinnamon Sauce (DF, GF) 99

Raspberry Ice Cream Sauce (DF, GF) 100

Strawberry Sauce (DF, GF) 101

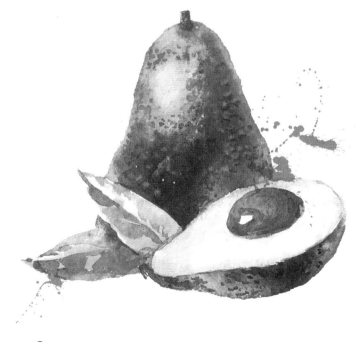

BONUS KETO SWEET EATS

I am delighted you have chosen my book to help you start or continue on your keto journey. Temptation by sweet treats can knock you off course so, to help you stay on the keto track, I am pleased to offer you three mini ebooks from my "Keto Sweet Eats Series," completely free of charge. These three mini ebooks cover how to make everything from keto chocolate cake to keto ice cream to keto fat bombs so you don't have to feel like you are missing out, whatever the occasion.

Simply visit the link below to get your free copy of all three mini ebooks ...

http://ketojane.com/saucebonus

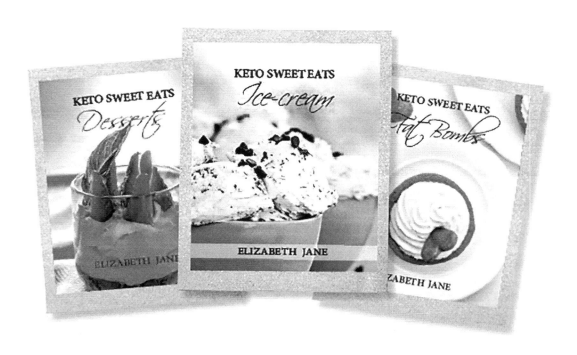

MUST-HAVE KETO SAUCE INGREDIENTS

Before you start heading to the kitchen to make these keto sauces, you may be wondering what are include as some of the go-to ingredients. While the sauces found in this book vary quite a bit, there are some ingredients that you may want to always have on hand. These include:

- Coconut aminos
- Olive oil
- Apple cider vinegar
- Balsamic vinegar
- White vinegar
- Garlic cloves
- Onions
- Garlic powder
- Onion powder
- Salt

- Ground black pepper
- Heavy cream
- Cream cheese
- Sour cream
- Mayonnaise
- Butter
- Shredded Parmesan cheese
- Lemons

Having these around the house will make putting these recipes together easy as they are staples that you will find throughout the recipes.

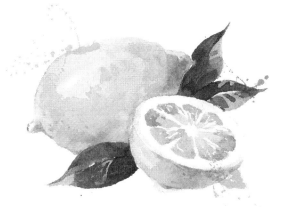

HOW TO STORE YOUR KETO SAUCES LIKE A PRO

When you are making these recipes, chances are you are going to have leftovers to use with other recipes, which is one of the many benefits of this cookbook. You can make a recipe and then have leftovers for at least a week! With that being said, you will want to know some tips and tricks for storing these sauces to help them maintain their freshness. Here are some tips that I can compiled through the years when making my own homemade keto sauces.

- Use glass Mason-style jars that are sealed tight and can be stored in the refrigerator easily.
- Use glass jars when storing your spice mixes to help them retain their flavor.
- If storing your spice mixes, be sure to keep them away from direct sunlight in a cool, dry place.

HOW THIS BOOK WORKS

This cookbook contains helpful cooking tips to help you get the best results possible. There are also serving suggestions included to give you an idea about what each of these recipes pairs well with.

You will also notice there are 5 symbols on the top right-hand side of each recipe. A key to these symbols is set out below:

Preparation Time:

Time required to prepare the recipe. This does not include the cooking time.

Cooking Time:

Time required to cook the recipe. This does not include the preparation time.

Servings:

How many servings each recipe requires. This can be adjusted. For example, by doubling the quantity of all of the ingredients, you can make twice as many servings.

Difficulty Level:

1: An easy-to-make recipe that can be put together with just a handful of ingredients and in a short amount of time.

2: These recipes are a little more difficult and time consuming but are still easy enough even for beginners!

3: A more advanced recipe for the adventurous cook! You will not see too many Level 3 recipes in this book. These recipes are ideal for when you have a little bit more time to spend in the kitchen and when you want to make something out of the ordinary.

Cost:

$: A low-budget everyday recipe.

$$: A moderately priced, middle-of-the-road recipe.

$$$: A more expensive recipe that is great for serving at a family gathering or party. These recipes tend to contain pricey ingredients.

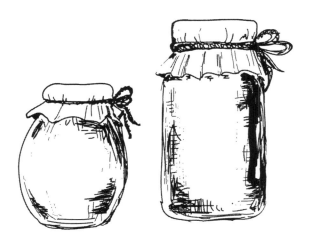

DIETARY LABELS

Within this book, you will notice that there are dietary labels. These will indicate whether a recipe is gluten-free, dairy-free, or vegetarian. Please note that many recipes can be made dairy-free by removing the cheese in them or by substituting the milk or cream for coconut milk. Each recipe will also be labeled if it is gluten-free. Although the majority of the recipes are gluten-free, always be sure to check the food label on the ingredients you buy due to the variations in certain product ingredients.

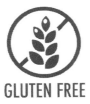
GLUTEN FREE

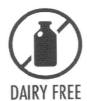
DAIRY FREE

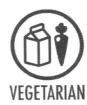
VEGETARIAN

You will also find a label indicating what each sauce recipes pairs well with, such as a vegetarian dish, meat-based dish, or a fish-based dish.

 = goes well with a vegetarian dish

 = goes well with a meat dish

 = goes well with a fish dish

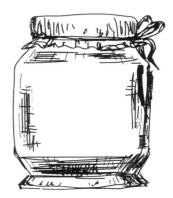

FINAL WORDS

Finally, I want to thank you for purchasing this book and I really hope it helps you keep to your health goals.

If you enjoyed this book or have any suggestions, then I'd appreciate it if you would leave a review or simply email me.

You can leave a review on Amazon at the link below, or email me at:
elizabeth@ketojane.com

To leave a review on Amazon, please visit:
http://ketojane.com/saucereview

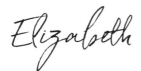

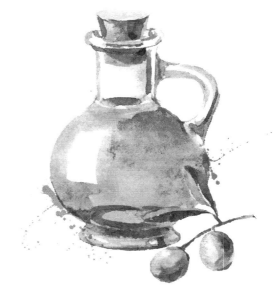

Sauces

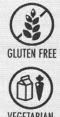

GLUTEN FREE

VEGETARIAN

QUICK AND EASY PESTO

Serves: 24

Difficulty Level: 1

Cost: $$

Prep Time: 5 minutes

Cook Time: 0 minutes

Calories: 67

Carbs: 1g

Fiber: 0g

Net Carbs: 1g

Protein: 1g

Fat: 7g

Calories from:
Carbs: 6%
Protein: 6%
Fat: 89%

Ingredients:

- ⅔ cup olive oil
- ¼ cup pine nuts
- ¼ cup cashews
- 2 cups packed fresh basil

- 2 garlic cloves, peeled and chopped
- Salt and pepper to taste

Directions:

1. Place all ingredients into a food processor and purée until a creamy pesto sauce forms.

2. Store covered in a sealed glass container in the fridge.

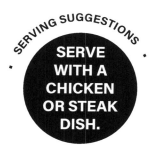

SERVING SUGGESTIONS

SERVE WITH A CHICKEN OR STEAK DISH.

GLUTEN FREE

Serves: 4

Difficulty Level: 1

Cost: $$

Prep Time: 10 minutes

Cook Time: 5-7 minutes

Calories: 167

Carbs: 2g

Fiber: 0g

Net Carbs: 2g

Protein: 7g

Fat: 15g

Calories from:
Carbs: 5%
Protein: 16%
Fat: 79%

CREAMY GARLIC CHEDDAR SAUCE

Ingredients:

- ¼ cup heavy cream
- ¼ cup cream cheese
- ¾ cup shredded cheddar cheese
- 2 garlic cloves, peeled and chopped
- 1 tsp. onion powder
- ½ tsp. paprika

Directions:

1. Place all ingredients into a stockpot over low-medium heat and whisk to combine.

2. Continue to whisk until the cheese melts.

3. Enjoy right away and store leftovers covered in the fridge.

SERVING SUGGESTIONS

SERVE OVER BROCCOLI OR BAKED CHICKEN

GLUTEN FREE

VEGETARIAN

Serves: 12

Difficulty Level: 1

Cost: $$

Prep Time: 10 minutes

Cook Time: 0 minutes

Calories: 16
Carbs: 3g
Fiber: 1g
Net Carbs: 2g
Protein: 1g
Fat: 1g

Calories from:
Carbs: 48%
Protein: 16%
Fat: 36%

MARINARA SAUCE

Ingredients:

* 28-ounce can peeled tomatoes (no sugar or salt added)
* 1 handful fresh basil
* 1 handful fresh parsley
* ½ sweet yellow onion, peeled and chopped
* 2 garlic cloves, peeled and chopped
* 1 Tbsp. Italian seasoning
* 1 tsp. sea salt
* ¼ tsp. ground black pepper

Directions:

1. Add the tomatoes to a food processor and purée until smooth.

2. Add in the remaining ingredients and blend together.

3. Enjoy right away and store leftovers in a sealed container in the fridge. You can also freeze the sauce for later use.

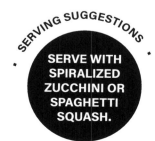

SERVING SUGGESTIONS

SERVE WITH SPIRALIZED ZUCCHINI OR SPAGHETTI SQUASH.

GLUTEN FREE

Serves: 12

Difficulty Level: 1

Cost: $$

Prep Time: 10 minutes

Cook Time: 10 minutes

Calories: 182
Carbs: 6g
Fiber: 2g
Net Carbs: 4g
Protein: 5g
Fat: 14g

Calories from:
Carbs: 14%
Protein: 12%
Fat: 74%

"PENNE" VODKA SAUCE

Ingredients:

- 1 cup heavy cream
- ½ cup butter
- 1 28-ounce can crushed tomatoes
- ½ cup unflavored vodka
- ½ sweet yellow onion, peeled and chopped
- 1 garlic clove, peeled and chopped
- 1 cup grated Parmesan cheese
- 1 Tbsp. Italian seasoning
- 1 tsp. sea salt
- ¼ tsp. ground black pepper

Directions:

1. Add the butter to a large skillet and heat until melted.

2. Add the onion, garlic, and vodka and cook for about 5 minutes.

3. Add the tomatoes and seasoning and stir well.

4. Add the heavy cream and cheese and stir until the cheese starts to melt.

5. Serve right away.

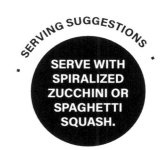

SERVING SUGGESTIONS

SERVE WITH SPIRALIZED ZUCCHINI OR SPAGHETTI SQUASH.

SWEET BUTTER SAUCE

GLUTEN FREE

Serves: 6

Difficulty Level: 1

Cost: $

Prep Time: 10 minutes

Cook Time: 8-10 minutes

Calories: 107

Carbs: 1g

Fiber: 0g

Net Carbs: 1g

Protein: 1g

Fat: 12g

Calories from:
Carbs: 3%
Protein: 3%
Fat: 93%

Ingredients:

- 5 Tbsp. salted butter
- ¼ cup heavy cream
- ¼ cup chicken or beef broth
- 1 tsp. garlic powder
- 1 tsp. onion powder
- ½ tsp. sea salt
- ⅛ tsp. ground black pepper
- 4-6 drops liquid stevia

Directions:

1. Add the butter to a saucepan over low-medium heat and brown the butter for about 3 minutes, swirling it around the pan frequently.

2. Add the butter to a stockpot with the remaining ingredients. Whisk to combine.

3. Simmer for 5-7 minutes.

4. Add the stevia and whisk again.

5. Enjoy right away.

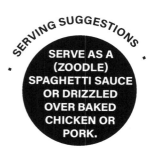

SERVING SUGGESTIONS

SERVE AS A (ZOODLE) SPAGHETTI SAUCE OR DRIZZLED OVER BAKED CHICKEN OR PORK.

GLUTEN FREE

Serves: 18

Difficulty Level: 1

Cost: $$

Prep Time: 10 minutes

Cook Time: 10 minutes

Calories: 97
Carbs: 1g
Fiber: 0g
Net Carbs: 1g
Protein: 4g
Fat: 9g

Calories from:
Carbs: 4%
Protein: 16%
Fat: 80%

ALFREDO PARMESAN SAUCE

Ingredients:

- ½ cup butter
- ½ cup heavy cream
- ½ cup grated Parmesan cheese
- ½ tsp. sea salt
- ⅛ tsp. ground black pepper

Directions:

1. Add the butter to a saucepan over low-medium heat and brown the butter for about 3 minutes, swirling it around the pan frequently.

2. Add the remaining ingredients and bring to a simmer.

3. Stir well until the cheese has melted into the mixture – cooking for about 7 minutes.

4. Enjoy right away.

SERVING SUGGESTIONS

SERVE AS A 'SPAGHETTI' SAUCE DRIZZLED OVER ANY MEAT DISH.

DAIRY FREE

GLUTEN FREE

Serves: 8

Difficulty Level: 1

Cost: $$

Prep Time: 10 minutes

Cook Time: 5 minutes

Calories: 303
Carbs: 8g
Fiber: 3g
Net Carbs: 5g
Protein: 7g
Fat: 30g

Calories from:
Carbs: 10%
Protein: 8%
Fat: 82%

ALMOND BUTTER SAUTÉ SAUCE

Ingredients:

- 1 cup unsweetened almond butter
- ½ cup olive oil
- ¼ cup coconut aminos
- 2 garlic cloves, peeled and chopped
- ½ tsp. sea salt

Directions:

1. Add all of the ingredients to a stockpot over low to medium heat and whisk.

2. Heat for about 5 minutes.

3. Remove from heat and serve right away.

  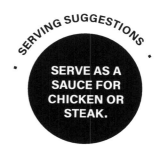

SERVING SUGGESTIONS

SERVE AS A SAUCE FOR CHICKEN OR STEAK.

GLUTEN FREE

Serves: 12

Difficulty Level: 1

Cost: $$

Prep Time: 10 minutes

Cook Time: 5 minutes

Calories: 82

Carbs: 1g

Fiber: 0g

Net Carbs: 1g

Protein: 1g

Fat: 9g

Calories from:
Carbs: 4%
Protein: 4%
Fat: 91%

DILL HOLLANDAISE SAUCE

Ingredients:

- ½ cup butter
- 3 egg yolks
- 1 Tbsp. freshly squeezed lemon juice
- 1 tsp. freshly chopped dill
- ½ tsp. salt
- ¼ tsp. crushed black pepper

Directions:

1. Add the butter to a saucepan over medium heat.

2. Add the remaining ingredients except the dill once the butter has melted and whisk well.

3. Add the dill and serve right away.

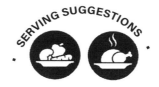

SERVING SUGGESTIONS

SERVE AS A SAUCE FOR VEGETABLES OR OMIT THE DILL AND ADD SOME TARRAGON AND WHITE WINE VINEGAR TO CREATE A BÉARNAISE SAUCE FOR STEAK.

GLUTEN FREE

Serves: 12

Difficulty Level: 1

Cost: $$

Prep Time: 10 minutes

Cook Time: 5-10 minutes

Calories: 32

Carbs: 1g

Fiber: 0g

Net Carbs: 1g

Protein: 0g

Fat: 3g

Calories from:
Carbs: 13%
Protein: 0%
Fat: 87%

SOUR CREAM AND ONION SAUCE

Ingredients:

- ½ cup sour cream
- 2 Tbsp. butter
- ½ cup water
- ½ white onion, peeled and diced
- 2 garlic cloves, peeled and chopped
- ½ tsp. sea salt

Directions:

1. Add the butter to a stockpot over medium heat. Add the onion and cook for 5 minutes or until translucent. Add the garlic and cook for another minute.

2. Add the remaining ingredients to a stockpot over low to medium heat and whisk.

3. Cook for 5-10 minutes, whisking until everything is combined.

4. Remove from the heat and use an immersion blender to purée the sauce until smooth.

5. Serve right away.

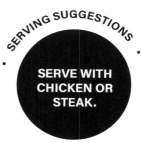

SERVING SUGGESTIONS

SERVE WITH CHICKEN OR STEAK.

GLUTEN FREE

Serves: 12

Difficulty Level: 1

Cost: $$

Prep Time: 10 minutes

Cook Time: 5-10 minutes

Calories: 73

Carbs: 1g

Fiber: 0g

Net Carbs: 1g

Protein: 4g

Fat: 6g

Calories from:
Carbs: 5%
Protein: 22%
Fat: 73%

CREAMY VEGETABLE SAUCE

Ingredients:

* 1 cup sour cream
* ½ cup shredded Parmesan cheese
* 1 Tbsp. freshly squeezed
* lemon juice
* 1 tsp. Italian seasoning
* ½ tsp. sea salt

Directions:

1. Add all of the ingredients to a stockpot over low to medium heat and whisk.

2. Warm for about 5 minutes, and then serve right away.

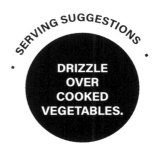

SERVING SUGGESTIONS

DRIZZLE OVER COOKED VEGETABLES.

Hot Sauces

DAIRY FREE

GLUTEN FREE

Serves: 25

Difficulty Level: 2

Cost: $

Prep Time: 10 minutes

Cook Time: 10 minutes

Calories: 9

Carbs: 1g

Fiber: 0g

Net Carbs: 1g

Protein: 0g

Fat: 1g

Calories from:
Carbs: 31%
Protein: 0%
Fat: 69%

TRADITIONAL HOT SAUCE

Ingredients:

- 1½ cups chopped tomatoes
- 1 Tbsp. olive oil
- ½ cup white vinegar
- 1 chili pepper, chopped
- ¼ white onion, peeled and chopped
- 1 garlic clove, peeled and chopped
- ½ tsp. cayenne pepper
- 1 tsp. onion powder
- ½ tsp. sea salt

Directions:

1. Heat a large stockpot over medium heat and add all the ingredients. Cook on medium for about 10 minutes until the tomatoes soften.

2. Use an immersion blender or food processor to purée the sauce until smooth.

3. Pass the sauce through a fine mesh strainer and pour into a sealed glass container.

4. Allow the sauce to completely cool before storing in the refrigerator.

SERVING SUGGESTIONS

ADD A ½ TSP. OR MORE TO ANY DISH THAT NEEDS A LITTLE EXTRA HEAT.

GLUTEN FREE

Serves: 25

Difficulty Level: 1

Cost: $

Prep Time: 10 minutes + chilling time

Cook Time: 0 minutes

Calories: 21

Carbs: 1g

Fiber: 0g

Net Carbs: 1g

Protein: 0g

Fat: 2g

Calories from:
Carbs: 18%
Protein: 0%
Fat: 82%

CREAMY JALAPEÑO HOT SAUCE

Ingredients:

- 2 Tbsp. butter
- 2 Tbsp. diced onion
- 1 small jalapeño pepper, seeded and chopped
- 1 celery stalk, chopped
- 1 cup sour cream
- 1 Tbsp. wasabi powder
- ½ tsp. salt

Directions:

1. Add the butter to a stockpot over medium heat. Add the onion, jalapeño pepper, and celery and cook for 5 minutes.

2. Remove from the heat and add to a food processor and pulse a few times.

3. Add the remaining ingredients to the food processor and purée until smooth.

4. Refrigerate for 1 hour before serving.

SERVING SUGGESTIONS

USE AS A VEGETABLE DIP OR TO HEAT UP A STEAK.

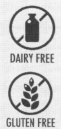

DAIRY FREE

GLUTEN FREE

Serves: 30

Difficulty Level: 1

Cost: $

Prep Time: 10 minutes

Cook Time: 0 minutes

Calories: 4
Carbs: 1g
Fiber: 0g
Net Carbs: 1g
Protein: 0g
Fat: 0g

Calories from:
Carbs: 100%
Protein: 0%
Fat: 0%

CURRY HOT PEPPER SAUCE

Ingredients:

- 5 jalapeño peppers, seeded and chopped
- 1 small red onion, peeled and chopped
- 3 garlic cloves, peeled and chopped
- ⅓ cup white vinegar
- Juice from 1 lime
- 1 tsp. curry powder
- 1 tsp. salt

Directions:

1. Place all ingredients into a high-speed blender or food processor and blend until smooth.

2. Store in the sealed glass container in the refrigerator until ready to serve.

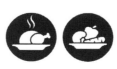 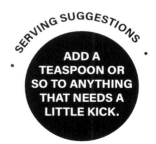

SERVING SUGGESTIONS

ADD A TEASPOON OR SO TO ANYTHING THAT NEEDS A LITTLE KICK.

31

DAIRY FREE

GLUTEN FREE

Serves: 30

Difficulty Level: 2

Cost: $

Prep Time: 10 minutes

Cook Time: 0 minutes

Calories: 70

Carbs: 11g

Fiber: 5g

Net Carbs: 6g

Protein: 2g

Fat: 3g

Calories from:
Carbs: 56%
Protein: 10%
Fat: 34%

CHILI PASTE

Ingredients:

- 1 pound chili peppers, chopped
- 1 small red onion, peeled and chopped
- 3 garlic cloves, peeled and chopped
- ⅓ cup olive oil
- 1 tsp. salt

Directions:

1. Add all of the ingredients except the olive oil and salt to a food processor and pulse until the garlic, onion, and peppers are chopped.

2. Preheat a medium skillet with the olive oil over low heat. Add the peppers, garlic, and onion.

3. Cook for about 15 minutes, stirring every couple of minutes.

4. Season with salt and then purée in a food processor again until smooth.

5. Store leftovers in a jar in the refrigerator.

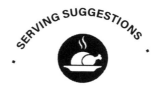

SERVING SUGGESTIONS

ADD A TEASPOON OR SO TO ANYTHING THAT NEEDS A LITTLE KICK. YOU CAN ALSO USE THIS SAUCE IN THAI-STYLE DISHES.

DAIRY FREE

GLUTEN FREE

Serves: 30

Difficulty Level: 2

Cost: $

Prep Time: 10 minutes

Cook Time: 0 minutes

Calories: 71
Carbs: 11g
Fiber: 5g
Net Carbs: 6g
Protein: 2g
Fat: 3g

Calories from:
Carbs: 56%
Protein: 10%
Fat: 34%

SPICY RED AND YELLOW PEPPER SAUCE

Ingredients:

- 1 pound chili peppers, chopped
- 1 red bell pepper, seeded and chopped
- 1 yellow bell pepper, seeded and chopped
- 3 garlic cloves, peeled and chopped
- ⅓ cup olive oil
- ½ tsp. black peppercorns, crushed
- 1 tsp. salt

Directions:

1. Add all ingredients to a food processor and blend until smooth. Add a tablespoon or two more of olive oil if you want a thinner sauce.

2. Store leftovers in a jar in the refrigerator.

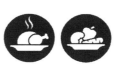

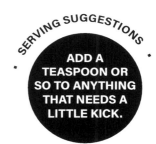

SERVING SUGGESTIONS

ADD A TEASPOON OR SO TO ANYTHING THAT NEEDS A LITTLE KICK.

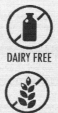

DAIRY FREE

GLUTEN FREE

SPICY TOMATO SAUCE

Serves: 8

Difficulty Level: 1

Cost: $

Prep Time: 10 minutes

Cook Time: 10 minutes

Calories: 11
Carbs: 2g
Fiber: 1g
Net Carbs: 1g
Protein: 1g
Fat: 0g

Calories from:
Carbs: 67%
Protein: 33%
Fat: 0%

Ingredients:

- 1 (14.5-ounce) can stewed tomatoes
- 1 small jalapeño pepper, seeded and chopped
- 2 garlic cloves, peeled and chopped
- 1 handful fresh basil, chopped
- 1 tsp. salt

Directions:

1. Add all the ingredients except the basil to a stockpot over medium heat. Bring to a boil and simmer for about 10 minutes.

2. Transfer the mixture along with the basil to a food processor and blend until smooth.

3. Enjoy right away and store leftovers in the fridge.

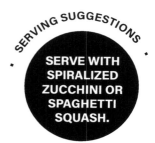

SERVING SUGGESTIONS

SERVE WITH SPIRALIZED ZUCCHINI OR SPAGHETTI SQUASH.

Dressings

BLUE CHEESE DRESSING

GLUTEN FREE

Serves: 12

Difficulty Level: 1

Cost: $

Prep Time: 10 minutes

Cook Time: 0 minutes

Calories: 126

Carbs: 5g

Fiber: 0g

Net Carbs: 5g

Protein: 2g

Fat: 11g

Calories from:
Carbs: 16%
Protein: 6%
Fat: 78%

Ingredients:

- ½ cup crumbled blue cheese
- ¾ cup full-fat sour cream
- ¼ cup whipped cream cheese
- ¾ cup olive oil-based mayonnaise
- 1 tsp. garlic powder
- 1 tsp. onion powder

Directions:

1. Add all ingredients to a food processor and purée until smooth.

2. Serve right away and store leftovers in a sealed container in the fridge.

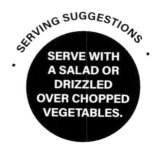

SERVING SUGGESTIONS

SERVE WITH A SALAD OR DRIZZLED OVER CHOPPED VEGETABLES.

GLUTEN FREE

Serves: 12

Difficulty Level: 1

Cost: $

Prep Time: 10 minutes

Cook Time: 0 minutes

Calories: 91

Carbs: 5g

Fiber: 0g

Net Carbs: 5g

Protein: 1g

Fat: 8g

Calories from:
Carbs: 21%
Protein: 4%
Fat: 75%

RANCH DRESSING

Ingredients:

- ½ cup full-fat sour cream
- ½ cup olive oil-based mayonnaise
- ¼ cup buttermilk
- 4 Tbsp. freshly squeezed lemon juice
- 1 tsp. garlic powder
- 1 tsp. onion powder
- 1 tsp. dried parsley
- 1 tsp. dried dill
- ⅛ tsp. ground black pepper

Directions:

1. Add all ingredients to a food processor and purée until smooth.

2. Serve right away and store leftovers in a sealed container in the fridge.

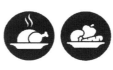

SERVING SUGGESTIONS

SERVE WITH A SALAD OR DRIZZLED OVER CHOPPED VEGETABLES.

CAESAR DRESSING

GLUTEN FREE

Serves: 8

Difficulty Level: 1

Cost: $

Prep Time: 10 minutes

Cook Time: 0 minutes

Calories: 91

Carbs: 4g

Fiber: 0g

Net Carbs: 4g

Protein: 4g

Fat: 7g

Calories from:
Carbs: 17%
Protein: 17%
Fat: 66%

Ingredients:

* 2 egg yolks
* ½ cup whipped cream cheese
* ½ cup olive oil-based mayonnaise
* 4 Tbsp. freshly squeezed lemon juice
* 1 teaspoon Worcestershire sauce
* 1 tsp. Dijon mustard
* 1 handful fresh parsley
* 2 Tbsp. grated Parmesan cheese
* ½ tsp. anchovy paste
* 2 tsp. garlic powder
* 1 tsp. onion powder

Directions:

1. Add all ingredients to a food processor and purée until smooth.

2. Serve right away and store leftovers in a sealed container in the fridge.

  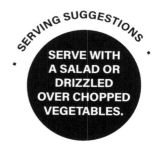

SERVING SUGGESTIONS

SERVE WITH A SALAD OR DRIZZLED OVER CHOPPED VEGETABLES.

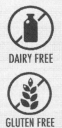

DAIRY FREE

GLUTEN FREE

Serves: 8

Difficulty Level: 1

Cost: $

Prep Time: 10 minutes

Cook Time: 0 minutes

Calories: 54
Carbs: 0g
Fiber: 0g
Net Carbs: 0g
Protein: 0g
Fat: 6g

Calories from:
Carbs: 0%
Protein: 0%
Fat: 100%

BALSAMIC VINAIGRETTE

Ingredients:

- ¼ cup olive oil
- ¼ cup balsamic vinegar
- ½ tsp. Italian seasoning
- ¼ tsp. sea salt

Directions:

1. Add all ingredients to a bowl and whisk to combine.

2. Pour into a sealed container and store on the counter.

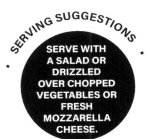

SERVING SUGGESTIONS

SERVE WITH A SALAD OR DRIZZLED OVER CHOPPED VEGETABLES OR FRESH MOZZARELLA CHEESE.

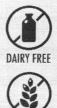

DAIRY FREE

GLUTEN FREE

Serves: 12

Difficulty Level: 1

Cost: $

Prep Time: 10 minutes

Cook Time: 0 minutes

Calories: 73
Carbs: 0g
Fiber: 0g
Net Carbs: 0g
Protein: 0g
Fat: 9g

Calories from:
Carbs: 0%
Protein: 0%
Fat: 100%

ITALIAN OLIVE OIL DRESSING

Ingredients:

- ½ cup olive oil
- ½ tsp. Italian seasoning
- 1 tsp. garlic powder
- ¼ tsp. sea salt

Directions:

1. Add all ingredients to a bowl and whisk to combine.
2. Pour into a sealed container and store on the counter.

SERVING SUGGESTIONS

SERVE WITH A SALAD OR DRIZZLED OVER CHOPPED VEGETABLES OR FRESH MOZZARELLA CHEESE.

GLUTEN FREE

Serves: 8

Difficulty Level: 1

Cost: $

Prep Time: 10 minutes

Cook Time: 0 minutes

Calories: 79

Carbs: 6g

Fiber: 2g

Net Carbs: 4g

Protein: 2g

Fat: 6g

Calories from:
Carbs: 28%
Protein: 9%
Fat: 63%

BASIL AVOCADO DRESSING

Ingredients:

- 1 cup of full-fat unsweetened Greek yogurt
- ¼ cup avocado oil (use can also use olive oil here)
- 1 avocado, pitted and sliced
- 1 handful fresh basil
- 1 tsp. garlic powder
- ¼ tsp. sea salt

Directions:

1. Add all ingredients into a food processor and blend until smooth.

2. Pour into a sealed container and store in the fridge.

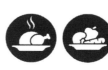

SERVING SUGGESTIONS

SERVE WITH A SALAD OR AS A DIP FOR VEGETABLES.

DAIRY FREE

GLUTEN FREE

LEMON HONEY MUSTARD DRESSING

Serves: 8

Difficulty Level: 1

Cost: $

Prep Time: 10 minutes

Cook Time: 0 minutes

Calories: 113
Carbs: 1g
Fiber: 0g
Net Carbs: 1g
Protein: 0g
Fat: 13g

Calories from:
Carbs: 3%
Protein: 0%
Fat: 97%

Ingredients:

- ½ cup olive oil
- 2 Tbsp. freshly squeezed lemon juice
- 2 Tbsp. Dijon mustard
- 1 Tbsp. raw honey
- 1 Tbsp. freshly chopped dill
- ¼ tsp. sea salt
- ⅛ tsp. ground black pepper

Directions:

1. Add all ingredients into a bowl and whisk.

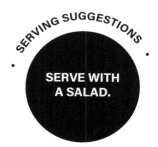

SERVING SUGGESTIONS

SERVE WITH A SALAD.

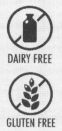

DAIRY FREE

GLUTEN FREE

Serves: 8

Difficulty Level: 1

Cost: $

Prep Time: 10 minutes

Cook Time: 0 minutes

Calories: 113
Carbs: 1g
Fiber: 0g
Net Carbs: 1g
Protein: 0g
Fat: 13g

Calories from:
Carbs: 3%
Protein: 0%
Fat: 97%

PARSLEY LEMON DRESSING

Ingredients:

- ½ cup olive oil
- ¼ cup freshly squeezed lemon juice
- 1 garlic clove, peeled and chopped
- 1 handful fresh parsley
- ¼ tsp. sea salt

Directions:

1. Add all ingredients to a food processor and blend until smooth.

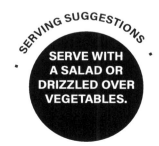

SERVING SUGGESTIONS

SERVE WITH A SALAD OR DRIZZLED OVER VEGETABLES.

43

Dips

GLUTEN FREE

Serves: 8
Difficulty Level: 1
Cost: $
Prep Time: 10 minutes + chilling time
Cook Time: 0 minutes

Calories: 46
Carbs: 2g
Fiber: 0g
Net Carbs: 2g
Protein: 0g
Fat: 4g

Calories from:
Carbs: 18%
Protein: 0%
Fat: 82%

SPICY MUSTARD DIPPING SAUCE

Ingredients:

- ¼ cup mayonnaise
- ¼ cup sour cream
- 1 tsp. Worcestershire sauce
- 1 Tbsp. spicy Dijon mustard
- ⅛ tsp. paprika
- ¼ tsp. cayenne pepper
- ¼ tsp. sea salt

Directions:

1. Add all ingredients to a mixing bowl and whisk well.

2. Chill in the refrigerator for 1 hour before serving.

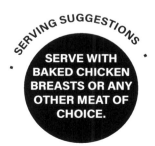

SERVING SUGGESTIONS

SERVE WITH BAKED CHICKEN BREASTS OR ANY OTHER MEAT OF CHOICE.

GLUTEN FREE

CLOVE AND BASIL MUSTARD SAUCE

Serves: 8

Difficulty Level: 1

Cost: $

Prep Time: 10 minutes + chilling time

Cook Time: 0 minutes

Calories: 60

Carbs: 4g

Fiber: 0g

Net Carbs: 4g

Protein: 0g

Fat: 5g

Calories from:
Carbs: 26%
Protein: 0%
Fat: 74%

Ingredients:

- ½ cup mayonnaise
- 1 Tbsp. spicy Dijon mustard
- ¼ tsp. ground cinnamon
- ⅛ tsp. ground cloves
- 1 handful fresh basil
- ¼ tsp. sea salt
- ⅛ tsp. ground black peppercorns

Directions:

1. Add all ingredients to a food processor and blend until smooth.

2. Chill in the refrigerator for 1 hour before serving.

SERVING SUGGESTIONS

SERVE WITH A SALAD FOR A WARM FALL OR WINTER FLAVOR OR SERVE AS A DIP FOR SAUTÉED OR GRILLED STEAK STRIPS.

BAKED BACON AND GARLIC DIP

GLUTEN FREE

Serves: 8

Difficulty Level: 2

Cost: $$

Prep Time: 15 minutes

Cook Time: 20-25 minutes

Calories: 165
Carbs: 2g
Fiber: 0g
Net Carbs: 2g
Protein: 7g
Fat: 15g

Calories from:
Carbs: 5%
Protein: 16%
Fat: 79%

Ingredients:

- 4 slices cooked bacon, chopped
- 1 cup full-fat whipped cream cheese
- ¼ cup ricotta cheese
- 2 garlic cloves, peeled and chopped
- 1 tsp. freshly chopped thyme
- 1 Tbsp. freshly chopped parsley
- ¼ tsp. sea salt
- Butter for greasing

Directions:

1. Preheat the oven to 350 degrees Fahrenheit and greasing 4 ramekins with butter.

2. Add all the ingredients to a mixing bowl and stir well.

3. Distribute the mixture evenly among the ramekin dishes and place on a baking sheet.

4. Bake for 20-25 minutes. Serve warm.

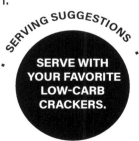

SERVING SUGGESTIONS

SERVE WITH YOUR FAVORITE LOW-CARB CRACKERS.

GLUTEN FREE

CARAMELIZED ONION CREAM CHEESE DIP

Serves: 8

Difficulty Level: 2

Cost: $$

Prep Time: 15 minutes

Cook Time: 10 minutes

Calories: 133

Carbs: 2g

Fiber: 0g

Net Carbs: 2g

Protein: 2g

Fat: 13g

Calories from:
Carbs: 6%
Protein: 6%
Fat: 88%

Ingredients:

* 1 cup full-fat whipped cream cheese
* ¼ tsp. nutmeg
* 1 tsp. freshly chopped rosemary
* ¼ tsp. sea salt
* 1 white onion, peeled and sliced thinly
* 2 Tbsp. butter

Directions:

1. Preheat a large skillet over medium heat with the butter.

2. Add the onions to the skillet and sauté until browned and caramelized. This may take 5-10 minutes. Be careful not to burn them as you just want them browned.

3. Add the cream cheese, nutmeg, rosemary, and salt to a mixing bowl and stir well to combine.

4. Transfer the cream cheese mixture to a serving bowl, and top with the caramelized onions.

SERVING SUGGESTIONS

SERVE WITH YOUR FAVORITE LOW-CARB CRACKERS.

GLUTEN FREE

Serves: 8

Difficulty Level: 1

Cost: $

Prep Time: 10 minutes + chilling time

Cook Time: 0 minutes

Calories: 68

Carbs: 3g

Fiber: 0g

Net Carbs: 3g

Protein: 1g

Fat: 6g

Calories from:
Carbs: 17%
Protein: 6%
Fat: 77%

SPICY CHILI PEPPER DIP

Ingredients:

- 1 cup full-fat sour cream
- 1 red jalapeño pepper, chopped
- 1 clove garlic, peeled and chopped
- 1 small onion, peeled and chopped
- ¼ tsp. sea salt
- Paprika for serving (optional for added heat)

Directions:

1. Add all ingredients minus the paprika to a food processor and purée until smooth.

2. Top with paprika, if desired, and chill for 1 hour before serving.

SERVING SUGGESTIONS

SERVE WITH YOUR FAVORITE LOW-CARB CRACKERS OR WITH STEAK OR BAKED CHICKEN BREAST.

CREAMY HERB DIP

GLUTEN FREE

Serves: 12

Difficulty Level: 1

Cost: $

Prep Time: 10 minutes + chilling time

Cook Time: 0 minutes

Calories: 101

Carbs: 2g

Fiber: 0g

Net Carbs: 2g

Protein: 4g

Fat: 9g

Calories from:
Carbs: 17%
Protein: 6%
Fat: 77%

Ingredients:

- 1 cup full-fat whipped cream cheese
- ½ cup full-fat ricotta cheese
- ½ cup shredded Parmesan cheese
- 2 green onions, chopped
- 1 Tbsp. freshly chopped dill
- 2 Tbsp. freshly chopped parsley
- 1 garlic clove, peeled and chopped
- 2 Tbsp. white onion diced
- ¼ tsp. sea salt

Directions:

1. Add all ingredients to a food processor and purée until smooth.

2. Chill for 1 hour before serving.

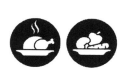

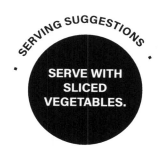

SERVING SUGGESTIONS

SERVE WITH SLICED VEGETABLES.

DAIRY FREE

GLUTEN FREE

Serves: 10

Difficulty Level: 1

Cost: $

Prep Time: 10 minutes

Cook Time: 0 minutes

Calories: 23

Carbs: 5g

Fiber: 1g

Net Carbs: 4g

Protein: 1g

Fat: 0g

Calories from:
Carbs: 83%
Protein: 17%
Fat: 0%

CRUSHED RED PEPPER AND GARLIC DIP

Ingredients:

- 1 cup no sugar-added tomato paste
- 2 garlic cloves, peeled and chopped
- 1 scallion, chopped
- 1 tsp. crushed red pepper flakes
- ¼ tsp. sea salt

Directions:

1. Add all ingredients minus to a food processor and purée until smooth.

2. Serve immediately or keep in the fridge in a sealed container.

SERVING SUGGESTIONS

SERVE WITH SLICED VEGETABLES. ALTERNATIVELY, YOU CAN USE THIS AS A MARINADE FOR MEAT DISHES.

GLUTEN FREE

Serves: 8

Difficulty Level: 1

Cost: $

Prep Time: 10 minutes

Cook Time: 0 minutes

Calories: 29

Carbs: 2g

Fiber: 0g

Net Carbs: 2g

Protein: 4g

Fat: 1g

Calories from:
Carbs: 24%
Protein: 48%
Fat: 27%

CRANBERRY COTTAGE CHEESE DIP

Ingredients:

* 1 cup fresh cranberries
* ¼ cup water
* 4-6 drops liquid stevia
* 1 cup full-fat cottage cheese
* ⅛ tsp. allspice

Directions:

1. Bring the water to a boil in a small saucepan.

2. Add the cranberries and simmer over medium heat for 10 minutes.

3. Allow the cranberries to cool. Add the stevia and stir well.

4. Add the cottage cheese and allspice to a mixing bowl and stir well.

5. Add to a serving bowl, top with cranberry sauce and enjoy.

SERVING SUGGESTIONS

SERVE WITH LOW-SUGAR FRUIT OR WITH YOUR FAVORITE LOW-CARB CRACKERS.

GLUTEN FREE

Serves: 8

Difficulty Level: 1

Cost: $

Prep Time: 10 minutes + chilling time

Cook Time: 0 minutes

Calories: 67

Carbs: 2g

Fiber: 0g

Net Carbs: 2g

Protein: 1g

Fat: 6g

Calories from:
Carbs: 12%
Protein: 6%
Fat: 82%

SOUR CREAM AND CUCUMBER DIP

Ingredients:

- 1 cup full-fat sour cream
- ½ cucumber, peeled and diced
- 1 Tbsp. freshly chopped dill
- 1 tsp. garlic powder
- ¼ tsp. salt

Directions:

1. Add all the ingredients to a mixing bowl and mix well.

2. Chill for 1 hour before serving.

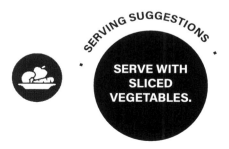

SERVING SUGGESTIONS

SERVE WITH SLICED VEGETABLES.

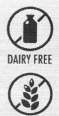

DAIRY FREE

GLUTEN FREE

Serves: 8

Difficulty Level: 1

Cost: $

Prep Time: 10 minutes + chilling time

Cook Time: 0 minutes

Calories: 211

Carbs: 10g

Fiber: 7g

Net Carbs: 3g

Protein: 2g

Fat: 20g

Calories from:
Carbs: 18%
Protein: 4%
Fat: 79%

GUACAMOLE

Ingredients:

* 4 ripe avocados pitted and cubed
* 1 small red onion, peeled and diced
* 1 handful fresh cilantro, chopped
* ¼ tsp. salt

Directions:

1. Add all the ingredients to a mixing bowl and mash.

2. Serve right away.

SERVING SUGGESTIONS

SERVE WITH SLICED VEGETABLES, WITH A SALAD OR WITH YOUR FAVORITE LOW-CARB CRACKERS.

DAIRY FREE

GLUTEN FREE

Serves: 18

Difficulty Level: 1

Cost: $

Prep Time: 10 minutes

Cook Time: 0 minutes

Calories: 72
Carbs: 4g
Fiber: 2g
Net Carbs: 2g
Protein: 1g
Fat: 7g

Calories from:
Carbs: 19%
Protein: 5%
Fat: 76%

SPICY GUACAMOLE

Ingredients:

- 3 ripe avocados, pitted and sliced
- 1 small red onion, peeled and diced
- 1 handful cilantro, chopped
- juice from 1 lemon
- 1 small jalapeño pepper, seeded and chopped
- ¼ tsp. cayenne pepper
- ½ tsp. salt

Directions:

1. Add the avocado, onion, and cilantro to a mixing bowl and mash.

2. Add the remaining ingredients and mix well.

3. Enjoy right away and refrigerate any leftovers.

SERVING SUGGESTIONS

SERVE WITH A SALAD OR WITH YOUR FAVORITE LOW-CARB CHIPS OR CRACKERS.

Condiments

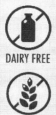

DAIRY FREE

GLUTEN FREE

Serves: 10

Difficulty Level: 1

Cost: $

Prep Time: 10 minutes

Cook Time: 0 minutes

Calories: 29
Carbs: 1g
Fiber: 1g
Net Carbs: 0g
Protein: 1g
Fat: 3g

Calories from:
Carbs: 11%
Protein: 11%
Fat: 77%

MAYONNAISE

Ingredients:

- ¾ cup avocado oil
- 1 tsp. white vinegar
- 2 egg yolks
- 2 tsp. Dijon mustard
- 1 tsp. garlic powder
- ¼ tsp. salt

Directions:

1. Add all the ingredients to a mixing bowl and, using an immersion blender, blend until creamy.

2. Store in the refrigerator.

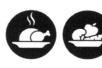

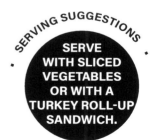

SERVING SUGGESTIONS

SERVE WITH SLICED VEGETABLES OR WITH A TURKEY ROLL-UP SANDWICH.

DAIRY FREE

GLUTEN FREE

Serves: 10

Difficulty Level: 1

Cost: $

Prep Time: 10 minutes

Cook Time: 0 minutes

Calories: 35
Carbs: 2g
Fiber: 1g
Net Carbs: 1g
Protein: 1g
Fat: 3g

Calories from:
Carbs: 21%
Protein: 10%
Fat: 69%

CHIPOTLE MAYONNAISE

Ingredients:

- ¾ cup avocado oil
- 1 tsp. white vinegar
- 2 egg yolks
- 2 tsp. Dijon mustard
- 2 chipotle chilis, seeded and chopped
- 1 Tbsp. adobo sauce
- 1 tsp. garlic powder
- ¼ tsp. salt

Directions:

1. Add all the ingredients to a mixing bowl and, using an immersion blender, blend until creamy.

2. Store in the refrigerator.

SERVING SUGGESTIONS

SERVE WITH SLICED VEGETABLES OR WITH A TURKEY ROLL-UP SANDWICH.

DAIRY FREE

GLUTEN FREE

Serves: 10

Difficulty Level: 1

Cost: $

Prep Time: 10 minutes

Cook Time: 0 minutes

Calories: 23
Carbs: 5g
Fiber: 1g
Net Carbs: 4g
Protein: 1g
Fat: 0g

Calories from:
Carbs: 83%
Protein: 17%
Fat: 0%

KETCHUP

Ingredients:

- 1 cup no sugar-added tomato paste
- ¼ cup white vinegar
- 2 Tbsp. water
- 1 garlic clove, peeled and chopped
- 2 Tbsp. onion powder
- ⅛ tsp. allspice
- ⅛ tsp. ground peppercorns
- 4-6 drops stevia
- ¼ tsp. salt

Directions:

1. Add all the ingredients to a food processor and blend until smooth.

2. Store in the refrigerator.

Serving Suggestions: Serve just as you would regular ketchup.

  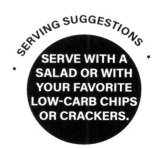

SERVING SUGGESTIONS
SERVE WITH A SALAD OR WITH YOUR FAVORITE LOW-CARB CHIPS OR CRACKERS.

DAIRY FREE

GLUTEN FREE

MUSTARD

Serves: 16

Difficulty Level: 1

Cost: $

Prep Time: 10 minutes

Cook Time: 0 minutes

Calories: 75

Carbs: 4g

Fiber: 2g

Net Carbs: 2g

Protein: 3g

Fat: 6g

Calories from:
Carbs: 20%
Protein: 15%
Fat: 66%

Ingredients:

- 1 cup mustard powder
- ¼ cup olive oil
- ¼ cup white wine vinegar
- ½ cup water
- 1 tsp. garlic powder
- 1 tsp. onion powder
- ⅛ tsp. freshly ground peppercorns
- ¼ tsp. salt

Directions:

1. Add all the ingredients to a mixing bowl and whisk well.

2. Store in the refrigerator.

SERVING SUGGESTIONS

SERVE JUST AS YOU WOULD REGULAR MUSTARD.

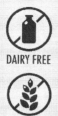

DAIRY FREE

GLUTEN FREE

Serves: 14

Difficulty Level: 1

Cost: $

Prep Time: 10 minutes

Cook Time: 0 minutes

Calories: 18

Carbs: 4g

Fiber: 1g

Net Carbs: 3g

Protein: 1g

Fat: 0g

Calories from:
Carbs: 80%
Protein: 20%
Fat: 0%

BBQ SAUCE

Ingredients:

- 1 cup no sugar-added tomato paste
- ¼ cup apple cider vinegar
- ¼ tsp. chili powder
- 1 tsp. paprika
- 1 tsp. garlic powder
- 1 tsp. onion powder
- ½ tsp. liquid smoke
- 4-6 drops stevia
- ¼ tsp. salt

Directions:

1. Add all the ingredients to a mixing bowl and, using an immersion blender, blend until smooth.

2. Store in the refrigerator.

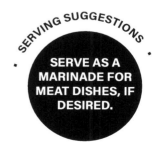

SERVING SUGGESTIONS

SERVE AS A MARINADE FOR MEAT DISHES, IF DESIRED.

Marinades

DAIRY FREE

GLUTEN FREE

Serves: 6

Difficulty Level: 1

Cost: $

Prep Time: 10 minutes

Cook Time: 0 minutes

Calories: 152

Carbs: 1g

Fiber: 0g

Net Carbs: 1g

Protein: 1g

Fat: 17g

Calories from:
Carbs: 2%
Protein: 2%
Fat: 95%

GRILLED CHICKEN MARINADE

Ingredients:

- ½ cup olive oil
- 3 Tbsp. coconut aminos
- ¼ cup apple cider vinegar
- 1 garlic clove, peeled and chopped
- ¼ tsp. chili powder
- 1 tsp. salt
- ½ tsp. ground black pepper

Directions:

1. Add all the ingredients to a mixing bowl and whisk.

2. Use as a marinade for chicken right away.

DAIRY FREE

GLUTEN FREE

Serves: 6

Difficulty Level: 1

Cost: $

Prep Time: 10 minutes

Cook Time: 0 minutes

Calories: 155

Carbs: 2g

Fiber: 0g

Net Carbs: 2g

Protein: 1g

Fat: 17g

Calories from:
Carbs: 5%
Protein: 2%
Fat: 93%

CARIBBEAN CHICKEN MARINADE

Ingredients:

- ½ cup olive oil
- ¼ cup fresh pineapple juice
- 3 Tbsp. coconut aminos
- 1 garlic clove, peeled and chopped
- ½ tsp. ground ginger
- 1 tsp. salt

Directions:

1. Add all the ingredients to a mixing bowl and whisk.

2. Use as a marinade for chicken right away.

DAIRY FREE

GLUTEN FREE

Serves: 6

Difficulty Level: 1

Cost: $

Prep Time: 10 minutes

Cook Time: 0 minutes

Calories: 154

Carbs: 2g

Fiber: 0g

Net Carbs: 2g

Protein: 1g

Fat: 17g

Calories from:
Carbs: 5%
Protein: 2%
Fat: 93%

SPICY CHICKEN MARINADE

Ingredients:

- ½ cup olive oil
- 2 Tbsp. apple cider vinegar
- 3 Tbsp. coconut aminos
- 2 garlic cloves, peeled and chopped
- 1 tsp. onion powder
- ½ tsp. ground ginger
- ¼ tsp. paprika
- 1 tsp. salt

Directions:

1. Add all the ingredients to a mixing bowl and whisk.

2. Use as a marinade for chicken right away.

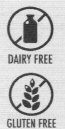

DAIRY FREE

GLUTEN FREE

Serves: 6

Difficulty Level: 1

Cost: $

Prep Time: 10 minutes

Cook Time: 0 minutes

Calories: 154

Carbs: 1g

Fiber: 0g

Net Carbs: 1g

Protein: 0g

Fat: 18g

Calories from:
Carbs: 2%
Protein: 2%
Fat: 96%

ITALIAN MARINADE

Ingredients:

- ½ cup olive oil
- 2 Tbsp. apple cider vinegar
- 1 garlic clove, peeled and chopped
- 1 Tbsp. chopped shallot
- 1 Tbsp. Italian seasoning
- 1 Tbsp. freshly chopped parsley
- 1 tsp. salt

Directions:

1. Add all the ingredients to a mixing bowl and whisk.

2. Use as a marinade for any poultry recipe.

DAIRY FREE

GLUTEN FREE

Serves: 6

Difficulty Level: 1

Cost: $

Prep Time: 10 minutes

Cook Time: 0 minutes

Calories: 54

Carbs: 3g

Fiber: 0g

Net Carbs: 3g

Protein: 1g

Fat: 5g

Calories from:
Carbs: 20%
Protein: 7%
Fat: 74%

JERK CHICKEN OR FISH MARINADE

Ingredients:

- 2 Tbsp. olive oil
- 2 Tbsp. white vinegar
- 2 Tbsp. coconut aminos
- ¼ cup fresh pineapple juice
- 1 garlic clove, peeled and chopped
- 1 green onion, chopped
- 1 tsp. allspice
- ½ tsp. nutmeg
- 1 tsp. ground ginger
- 1 tsp. salt

Directions:

1. Add all the ingredients to a food processor and purée until smooth.

2. Use as a marinade for a chicken or fish recipe.

DAIRY FREE

GLUTEN FREE

Serves: 4

Difficulty Level: 1

Cost: $

Prep Time: 10 minutes

Cook Time: 0 minutes

Calories: 133
Carbs: 2g
Fiber: 1g
Net Carbs: 2g
Protein: 1g
Fat: 14g

Calories from:
Carbs: 6%
Protein: 3%
Fat: 91%

MEDITERRANEAN MARINADE

Ingredients:

- 4 Tbsp. olive oil
- Juice from 1 lemon
- 1 garlic clove, peeled and chopped
- 1 tsp. cumin
- 2 tsp. coriander
- 1 handful fresh parsley, chopped
- 1 tsp. salt
- ¼ tsp. ground black pepper

Directions:

1. Add all the ingredients to a food processor and purée until smooth.

2. Use as a marinade for a chicken or fish recipe.

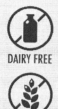

DAIRY FREE

GLUTEN FREE

Serves: 6

Difficulty Level: 1

Cost: $

Prep Time: 10 minutes

Cook Time: 0 minutes

Calories: 151

Carbs: 1g

Fiber: 0g

Net Carbs: 1g

Protein: 0g

Fat: 17g

Calories from:
Carbs: 3%
Protein: 0%
Fat: 97%

LEMON AND HERB MARINADE

Ingredients:

- ½ cup olive oil
- Juice from 1 lemon
- 1 Tbsp. freshly chopped dill
- 1 tsp. freshly chopped thyme
- 1 garlic clove, chopped
- 1 tsp. cumin
- 1 tsp. salt
- ¼ tsp. ground black pepper

Directions:

1. Add all the ingredients to a mixing bowl and whisk.

2. Use as a marinade for a chicken or fish recipe.

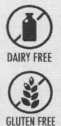

DAIRY FREE

GLUTEN FREE

Serves: 6

Difficulty Level: 1

Cost: $

Prep Time: 10 minutes

Cook Time: 0 minutes

Calories: 156
Carbs: 2g
Fiber: 0g
Net Carbs: 2g
Protein: 1g
Fat: 17g

Calories from:
Carbs: 5%
Protein: 2%
Fat: 93%

CLASSIC STEAK MARINADE

Ingredients:

- ½ cup olive oil
- ¼ cup coconut aminos
- Juice from 1 lemon
- 1 tsp. garlic powder
- 1 tsp. onion powder
- 1 tsp. crushed red pepper flakes
- 1 tsp. salt
- ¼ tsp. ground black pepper

Directions:

1. Add all the ingredients to a mixing bowl and whisk.

2. Use as a marinade for a steak or any other red meat recipe.

DAIRY FREE

GLUTEN FREE

Serves: 3

Difficulty Level: 1

Cost: $

Prep Time: 10 minutes

Cook Time: 0 minutes

Calories: 90
Carbs: 2g
Fiber: 0g
Net Carbs: 2g
Protein: 1g
Fat: 9g

Calories from:
Carbs: 9%
Protein: 4%
Fat: 87%

BALSAMIC AND MUSTARD STEAK MARINADE

Ingredients:

- 2 Tbsp. olive oil
- 1 Tbsp. balsamic vinegar
- 1 Tbsp. coconut aminos
- 1 tsp. Dijon mustard
- 1 garlic clove, peeled and chopped
- 1 tsp. onion powder
- 1 tsp. salt
- ¼ tsp. ground black pepper

Directions:

1. Add all the ingredients to a mixing bowl and whisk.

2. Use as a marinade for a steak or any other red meat recipe.

DAIRY FREE

GLUTEN FREE

Serves: 6

Difficulty Level: 1

Cost: $

Prep Time: 10 minutes

Cook Time: 0 minutes

Calories: 23

Carbs: 5g

Fiber: 0g

Net Carbs: 5g

Protein: 1g

Fat: 0g

Calories from:
Carbs: 83%
Protein: 17%
Fat: 0%

TERIYAKI MARINADE

Ingredients:

- ½ cup coconut aminos
- ⅓ cup water
- 1 garlic clove, chopped
- 1 Tbsp. raw honey
- ½ tsp. ground cinnamon

Directions:

1. Add all the ingredients to a mixing bowl and whisk.

2. Use as a marinade for any meat based recipe.

Butter Marinades

GLUTEN FREE

Serves: 6

Difficulty Level: 1

Cost: $

Prep Time: 10 minutes

Cook Time: 0 minutes

Calories: 139
Carbs: 1g
Fiber: 0g
Net Carbs: 1g
Protein: 0g
Fat: 15g

Calories from:
Carbs: 3%
Protein: 0%
Fat: 97%

DILL AND BUTTER MARINADE

Ingredients:

- ½ cup butter, softened
- 1 garlic clove, peeled and chopped
- 1 green onion, chopped
- 1 Tbsp. freshly chopped dill
- ½ tsp. salt

Directions:

1. Add all the ingredients to a food processor and purée until smooth.

2. Use as a marinade for a steak or chicken recipe.

GLUTEN FREE

Serves: 6

Difficulty Level: 1

Cost: $

Prep Time: 10 minutes

Cook Time: 0 minutes

Calories: 137
Carbs: 0g
Fiber: 0g
Net Carbs: 0g
Protein: 0g
Fat: 15g

Calories from:
Carbs: 0%
Protein: 0%
Fat: 100%

GARLIC AND CHIVE MARINADE

Ingredients:

- ½ cup butter, softened
- 2 garlic cloves, peeled and chopped
- 2 Tbsp. chopped chives
- ½ tsp. salt

Directions:

1. Add all the ingredients to a food processor and purée until smooth.

2. Use as a marinade for a steak or chicken recipe.

HERBED BUTTER MARINADE

GLUTEN FREE

Serves: 6

Difficulty Level: 1

Cost: $

Prep Time: 10 minutes

Cook Time: 0 minutes

Calories: 138

Carbs: 1g

Fiber: 0g

Net Carbs: 1g

Protein: 0g

Fat: 15g

Calories from:
Carbs: 3%
Protein: 0%
Fat: 97%

Ingredients:

- ½ cup butter, softened
- 2 garlic cloves, peeled and chopped
- 1 tsp. freshly chopped thyme
- 1 tsp. freshly chopped parsley
- 1 tsp. freshly chopped rosemary
- ½ tsp. salt

Directions:

1. Add all the ingredients to a food processor and purée until smooth.

2. Use as a marinade for a steak, chicken, or turkey recipe.

STEAK BUTTER MARINADE

GLUTEN FREE

Serves: 6

Difficulty Level: 1

Cost: $

Prep Time: 10 minutes

Cook Time: 0 minutes

Calories: 139

Carbs: 1g

Fiber: 0g

Net Carbs: 1g

Protein: 0g

Fat: 15g

Calories from:
Carbs: 3%
Protein: 0%
Fat: 97%

Ingredients:

- ½ cup butter, softened
- 2 garlic cloves, peeled and chopped
- 2 tsp. Worcestershire sauce
- 1 tsp. salt
- ¼ tsp. ground black pepper

Directions:

1. Add all the ingredients to a food processor and purée until smooth.

2. Use as a marinade for steak.

GLUTEN FREE

Serves: 6

Difficulty Level: 1

Cost: $

Prep Time: 10 minutes

Cook Time: 0 minutes

Calories: 110

Carbs: 1g

Fiber: 0g

Net Carbs: 1g

Protein: 0g

Fat: 12g

Calories from:
Carbs: 4%
Protein: 0%
Fat: 96%

OLIVE OIL AND BUTTER SHRIMP MARINADE

Ingredients:

- ¼ cup butter, softened
- 2 Tbsp. olive oil
- 2 garlic cloves, peeled and chopped
- 1 tsp. shallot peeled and shallot
- ½ tsp. salt
- ¼ tsp. ground black pepper

Directions:

1. Add all the ingredients to a food processor and purée until smooth.

2. Use as a marinade for shrimp or any other fish recipe.

Seasonings and Rubs

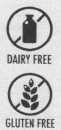

DAIRY FREE

GLUTEN FREE

Serves: 8

Difficulty Level: 1

Cost: $

Prep Time: 10 minutes

Cook Time: 0 minutes

Calories: 5

Carbs: 1g

Fiber: 0g

Net Carbs: 1g

Protein: 0g

Fat: 0g

Calories from:
Carbs: 100%
Protein: 0%
Fat: 0%

CLASSIC ITALIAN SEASONING

Ingredients:

- 1 Tbsp. dried oregano
- 1 Tbsp. dried parsley
- 1 Tsp. dried thyme
- 1 tsp. onion powder
- 1 tsp garlic powder
- ½ tsp. salt
- ¼ tsp. ground black pepper

Directions:

1. Add all the ingredients to a mixing bowl and mix well.

   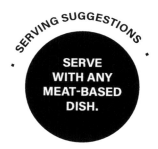

SERVING SUGGESTIONS

SERVE WITH ANY MEAT-BASED DISH.

DAIRY FREE

GLUTEN FREE

Serves: 8

Difficulty Level: 1

Cost: $

Prep Time: 10 minutes

Cook Time: 0 minutes

Calories: 6
Carbs: 1g
Fiber: 0g
Net Carbs: 1g
Protein: 0g
Fat: 0g

Calories from:
Carbs: 100%
Protein: 0%
Fat: 0%

TACO SEASONING

Ingredients:

- 1 Tbsp. dried oregano
- 1 tsp. cumin
- 1 tsp. coriander
- ½ tsp. paprika
- ½ tsp. chili powder
- 1 tsp. onion powder
- 1 tsp garlic powder
- ½ tsp. salt

Directions:

1. Add all the ingredients to a mixing bowl and mix well.

SERVING SUGGESTIONS

SERVE WITH A TURKEY OR BEEF TACO RECIPE.

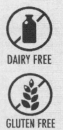

DAIRY FREE

GLUTEN FREE

FAJITA SEASONING

Serves: 8

Difficulty Level: 1

Cost: $

Prep Time: 10 minutes

Cook Time: 0 minutes

Calories: 11
Carbs: 2g
Fiber: 1g
Net Carbs: 1g
Protein: 0g
Fat: 0g

Calories from:
Carbs: 100%
Protein: 0%
Fat: 0%

Ingredients:

- 1 Tbsp. chili powder
- 1 tsp. paprika
- 1 Tbsp. onion powder
- 1 Tbsp. garlic powder
- ½ tsp. cayenne pepper
- ½ tsp. salt

Directions:

1. Add all the ingredients to a mixing bowl and mix well.

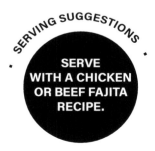

SERVING SUGGESTIONS

SERVE WITH A CHICKEN OR BEEF FAJITA RECIPE.

DAIRY FREE

GLUTEN FREE

Serves: 8

Difficulty Level: 1

Cost: $

Prep Time: 10 minutes

Cook Time: 0 minutes

Calories: 8
Carbs: 2g
Fiber: 0g
Net Carbs: 2g
Protein: 0g
Fat: 0g

Calories from:
Carbs: 100%
Protein: 0%
Fat: 0%

SEASONED SALT RUB

Ingredients:

* 1 Tbsp. onion powder
* 1 Tbsp. garlic powder
* 1 tsp. chili powder
* 1 Tbsp. dried parsley
* 1 Tbsp. sea salt
* ½ tsp. ground black pepper

Directions:

1. Add all the ingredients to a mixing bowl and mix well.

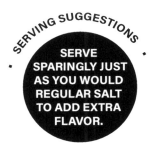

SERVING SUGGESTIONS

SERVE SPARINGLY JUST AS YOU WOULD REGULAR SALT TO ADD EXTRA FLAVOR.

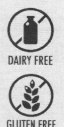

DAIRY FREE

GLUTEN FREE

Serves: 8

Difficulty Level: 1

Cost: $

Prep Time: 10 minutes

Cook Time: 0 minutes

Calories: 7
Carbs: 2g
Fiber: 0g
Net Carbs: 2g
Protein: 0g
Fat: 0g

Calories from:
Carbs: 100%
Protein: 0%
Fat: 0%

RANCH SEASONING

Ingredients:

* 1 Tbsp. dried parsley
* 1 Tbsp. dried dill
* 1 Tbsp. garlic powder
* 2 tsp. onion powder
* 1 Tbsp. buttermilk powder
* 1 tsp. salt
* ½ tsp. ground black pepper

Directions:

1. Add all the ingredients to a mixing bowl and mix well.

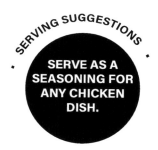

SERVING SUGGESTIONS

SERVE AS A SEASONING FOR ANY CHICKEN DISH.

DAIRY FREE

GLUTEN FREE

CURRY POWDER

Serves: 8

Difficulty Level: 1

Cost: $

Prep Time: 10 minutes

Cook Time: 0 minutes

Calories: 6

Carbs: 1g

Fiber: 1g

Net Carbs: 0g

Protein: 0g

Fat: 0g

Calories from:
Carbs: 100%
Protein: 0%
Fat: 0%

Ingredients:

- 1 tsp. paprika
- 1 tsp. cumin
- 1 tsp. ground cardamom
- ¼ cup turmeric
- 1 tsp. ground cinnamon
- 1 tsp. coriander
- 1 tsp. mustard powder
- 1 tsp. cayenne pepper
- 1 tsp. salt

Directions:

1. Add all the ingredients to a mixing bowl and mix well.

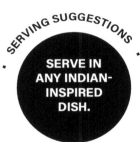

SERVING SUGGESTIONS

SERVE IN ANY INDIAN-INSPIRED DISH.

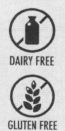

DAIRY FREE

GLUTEN FREE

Serves: 8

Difficulty Level: 1

Cost: $

Prep Time: 10 minutes

Cook Time: 0 minutes

Calories: 10

Carbs: 2g

Fiber: 1g

Net Carbs: 1g

Protein: 0g

Fat: 0g

Calories from:
Carbs: 100%
Protein: 0%
Fat: 0%

CHILI POWDER

Ingredients:

- 1 Tbsp. chili powder
- 1 tsp. paprika
- 1 tsp. cumin
- 1 Tbsp. garlic powder
- 1 tsp. onion powder
- 1 tsp. dried oregano
- ¼ tsp. cayenne pepper
- 1 tsp. salt

Directions:

1. Add all the ingredients to a mixing bowl and mix well.

SERVING SUGGESTIONS

SERVE WITH ANY DISH TO ADD EXTRA HEAT.

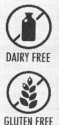

DAIRY FREE

GLUTEN FREE

Serves: 8

Difficulty Level: 1

Cost: $

Prep Time: 10 minutes

Cook Time: 0 minutes

Calories: 7

Carbs: 1g

Fiber: 1g

Net Carbs: 0g

Protein: 0g

Fat: 0g

Calories from:
Carbs: 100%
Protein: 0%
Fat: 0%

ADOBO SEASONING

Ingredients:

- 1 Tbsp. dried oregano
- 1 tsp. cumin
- 1 Tsp. garlic powder
- 1 tsp. onion powder
- 1 tsp. chili powder
- 1 tsp. paprika
- 1 tsp. salt

Directions:

1. Add all the ingredients to a mixing bowl and mix well.

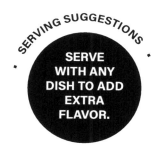

SERVING SUGGESTIONS

SERVE WITH ANY DISH TO ADD EXTRA FLAVOR.

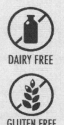

DAIRY FREE

GLUTEN FREE

Serves: 8

Difficulty Level: 1

Cost: $

Prep Time: 10 minutes

Cook Time: 0 minutes

Calories: 4
Carbs: 1g
Fiber: 0g
Net Carbs: 1g
Protein: 0g
Fat: 0g

Calories from:
Carbs: 100%
Protein: 0%
Fat: 0%

BLACKENED SEASONING

Ingredients:

- 1 tsp. paprika
- 1 Tbsp. garlic powder
- 1 Tbsp. onion powder
- 1 Tbsp. dried thyme
- ¼ tsp. cayenne pepper
- 1 tsp. dried oregano
- 1 tsp. salt
- ¼ tsp. ground black pepper

Directions:

1. Add all the ingredients to a mixing bowl and mix well.

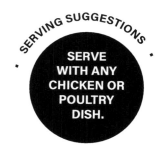

SERVING SUGGESTIONS

SERVE WITH ANY CHICKEN OR POULTRY DISH.

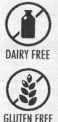

DAIRY FREE

GLUTEN FREE

Serves: 8

Difficulty Level: 1

Cost: $

Prep Time: 10 minutes

Cook Time: 0 minutes

Calories: 4
Carbs: 1g
Fiber: 1g
Net Carbs: 0g
Protein: 0g
Fat: 0g

Calories from:
Carbs: 100%
Protein: 0%
Fat: 0%

PUMPKIN SPICE SEASONING

Ingredients:

* 3 tsp. ground cinnamon
* 2 tsp. ground ginger
* 1 tsp. ground nutmeg
* 1 tsp. allspice
* 1 tsp. ground cloves

Directions:

1. Add all the ingredients to a mixing bowl and mix well.

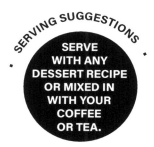

SERVING SUGGESTIONS

SERVE WITH ANY DESSERT RECIPE OR MIXED IN WITH YOUR COFFEE OR TEA.

Glazes and Infused Oils

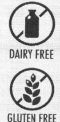

DAIRY FREE

GLUTEN FREE

Serves: 24

Difficulty Level: 2

Cost: $$

Prep Time: 10 minutes

Cook Time: 6 minutes

Calories: 73
Carbs: 0g
Fiber: 0g
Net Carbs: 0g
Protein: 0g
Fat: 8g

Calories from:
Carbs: 0%
Protein: 0%
Fat: 100%

GARLIC AND THYME OIL

Ingredients:

* 1 cup extra virgin olive oil
* 4 garlic cloves, peeled
* 2 thyme sprigs

Directions:

1. Add the olive oil and garlic to a saucepan over medium to high heat and bring to a boil.

2. Lower the heat and bring to a simmer. Simmer for about 6 minutes.

3. Remove the garlic and chop.

4. Place the garlic into the base of a glass jar and pour the olive oil over the top.

5. Add the thyme sprigs.

6. Allow the oil to cool before placing the cap on the oil.

   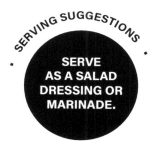

SERVING SUGGESTIONS

SERVE AS A SALAD DRESSING OR MARINADE.

DAIRY FREE

GLUTEN FREE

GARLIC AND ROSEMARY OIL

Serves: 24

Difficulty Level: 2

Cost: $$

Prep Time: 10 minutes

Cook Time: 6 minutes

Calories: 74

Carbs: 0g

Fiber: 0g

Net Carbs: 0g

Protein: 0g

Fat: 8g

Calories from:
Carbs: 0%
Protein: 0%
Fat: 100%

Ingredients:

* 1 cup extra virgin olive oil
* 4 garlic cloves, peeled
* 2 rosemary, sprigs

Directions:

1. Add the olive oil and garlic to a saucepan over medium to high heat and bring to a boil.

2. Lower the heat and bring to a simmer. Simmer for about 6 minutes.

3. Remove the garlic and chop.

4. Place the garlic into the base of a glass jar and pour the olive oil over the top.

5. Add the rosemary sprigs.

6. Allow the oil to cool before placing the cap on the oil.

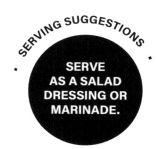

SERVING SUGGESTIONS

SERVE AS A SALAD DRESSING OR MARINADE.

DAIRY FREE

GLUTEN FREE

Serves: 12

Difficulty Level: 1

Cost: $$

Prep Time: 10 minutes

Cook Time: 0 minutes

Calories: 15

Carbs: 1g

Fiber: 0g

Net Carbs: 1g

Protein: 0g

Fat: 1g

Calories from:
Carbs: 31%
Protein: 0%
Fat: 69%

GINGER CHICKEN GLAZE

Ingredients:

- ¼ cup coconut aminos
- 1 Tbsp. melted coconut oil
- 2 garlic cloves, peeled and chopped
- 1 Tbsp. freshly grated ginger
- 1 tsp. sea salt
- ¼ tsp. ground black pepper

Directions:

1. Add all ingredients to a mixing bowl and whisk to combine.

2. Use as a glaze for chicken or other poultry dishes.

SERVING SUGGESTIONS

USE AS A GLAZE FOR CHICKEN BREASTS, OR CHICKEN WINGS.

DAIRY FREE

GLUTEN FREE

Serves: 3

Difficulty Level: 1

Cost: $$

Prep Time: 10 minutes

Cook Time: 0 minutes

Calories: 48

Carbs: 1g

Fiber: 0g

Net Carbs: 1g

Protein: 1g

Fat: 5g

Calories from:
Carbs: 8%
Protein: 8%
Fat: 85%

BALSAMIC STEAK GLAZE

Ingredients:

- 2 Tbsp. balsamic vinegar
- 1 Tbsp. coconut aminos
- 1 Tbsp. olive oil
- 2 garlic cloves, peeled and chopped
- ¼ tsp. ground black pepper

Directions:

1. Add all ingredients to a mixing bowl and whisk to combine.

2. Use as a glaze for steak dishes.

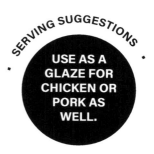

SERVING SUGGESTIONS

USE AS A GLAZE FOR CHICKEN OR PORK AS WELL.

GLUTEN FREE

Serves: 3

Difficulty Level: 1

Cost: $$

Prep Time: 10 minutes

Cook Time: 5 minutes

Calories: 73

Carbs: 1g

Fiber: 0g

Net Carbs: 1g

Protein: 0g

Fat: 8g

Calories from:
Carbs: 5%
Protein: 0%
Fat: 95%

BUTTER STEAK GLAZE

Ingredients:

- 2 Tbsp. salted butter
- 1 Tbsp. balsamic vinegar
- 2 garlic cloves, peeled and chopped
- 1 tsp. shallots, peeled and chopped

Directions:

1. Add all ingredients to a stockpot over low to medium heat and cook to brown the butter.

2. Whisk well and then serve right away.

SERVING SUGGESTIONS

USE AS A GLAZE FOR STEAK DISHES. YOU CAN ALSO USE THIS AS A SAUCE FOR BURGERS

Dessert Sauces

CARAMEL SAUCE

GLUTEN FREE

Serves: 14

Difficulty Level: 1

Cost: $$

Prep Time: 5 minutes

Cook Time: 12 minutes

Calories: 79

Carbs: 0g

Fiber: 0g

Net Carbs: 0g

Protein: 0g

Fat: 9g

Calories from:
Carbs: 5%
Protein: 0%
Fat: 95%

Ingredients:

* ½ cup salted butter
* ⅔ cup heavy cream
* 1 tsp. pure vanilla extract

Directions:

1. Add the butter to a stockpot over low to medium heat and cook for about 2 minutes or until the butter has browned.

2. Add in the remaining ingredients and stir to combine. Bring to a simmer and simmer for about 10 minutes until the mixture forms a caramel-like sticky consistency.

3. Serve while warm and store leftovers in the fridge.

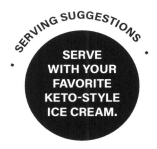

SERVING SUGGESTIONS

SERVE WITH YOUR FAVORITE KETO-STYLE ICE CREAM.

HOT FUDGE SAUCE

GLUTEN FREE

Serves: 22

Difficulty Level: 1

Cost: $$

Prep Time: 10 minutes

Cook Time: 10 minutes

Calories: 109

Carbs: 6g

Fiber: 2g

Net Carbs: 4g

Protein: 1g

Fat: 11g

Calories from:
Carbs: 19%
Protein: 3%
Fat: 78%

Ingredients:

- ½ cup butter
- ½ cup unsweetened cocoa powder
- ½ cup unsweetened dark chocolate chips
- ¼ cup erythritol
- 1 cup heavy cream
- ½ cup full-fat coconut milk

Directions:

1. Add all the ingredients to a stockpot over low to medium heat and continually stir until the chocolate is melted completely.

2. Serve while warm and store leftovers in the fridge.

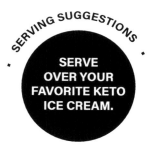

SERVING SUGGESTIONS

SERVE OVER YOUR FAVORITE KETO ICE CREAM.

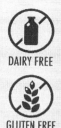

DAIRY FREE

GLUTEN FREE

Serves: 10

Difficulty Level: 1

Cost: $

Prep Time: 5 minutes

Cook Time: 10 minutes

Calories: 32
Carbs: 9g
Fiber: 1g
Net Carbs: 8g
Protein: 0g
Fat: 0g

Calories from:
Carbs: 100%
Protein: 0%
Fat: 0%

APPLE CINNAMON SAUCE

Ingredients:

* 2 apples peeled, cored, and sliced
* 1 Tbsp. ground cinnamon
* 1 Tbsp. water
* 1 tsp. pure vanilla extract
* 1 Tbsp. raw honey

Directions:

1. Add all ingredients to a stockpot and bring to a simmer.

2. Simmer for 10 minutes or until the apples are soft.

3. Transfer to a food processor or use an immersion blender and blend until smooth.

4. Store in the refrigerator until ready to serve.

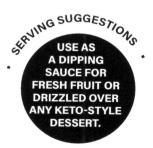

SERVING SUGGESTIONS

USE AS A DIPPING SAUCE FOR FRESH FRUIT OR DRIZZLED OVER ANY KETO-STYLE DESSERT.

DAIRY FREE

GLUTEN FREE

Serves: 12

Difficulty Level: 1

Cost: $

Prep Time: 5 minutes

Cook Time: 15 minutes

Calories: 11
Carbs: 8g
Fiber: 1g
Net Carbs: 7g
Protein: 0g
Fat: 0g

Calories from:
Carbs: 100%
Protein: 0%
Fat: 0%

RASPBERRY ICE CREAM SAUCE

Ingredients:

- 2 cups fresh raspberries
- 1 cup water
- ¼ cup erythritol

Directions:

1. Add all ingredients to a stockpot and bring to a simmer. Simmer for 15 minutes, mashing the raspberries throughout the cook time.

2. Strain the syrup through a fine mesh strainer and store in the refrigerator until ready to use.

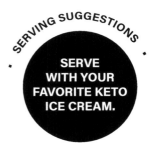

SERVING SUGGESTIONS

SERVE WITH YOUR FAVORITE KETO ICE CREAM.

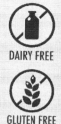

DAIRY FREE

GLUTEN FREE

Serves: 12

Difficulty Level: 1

Cost: $

Prep Time: 5 minutes

Cook Time: 15 minutes

Calories: 8
Carbs: 7g
Fiber: 1g
Net Carbs: 6g
Protein: 0g
Fat: 0g

Calories from:
Carbs: 100%
Protein: 0%
Fat: 0%

STRAWBERRY SAUCE

Ingredients:

- 2 cups fresh strawberries
- 1 cup water
- ¼ cup erythritol

Directions:

1. Add all ingredients to a stockpot and bring to a simmer. Simmer for 15 minutes, mashing the strawberries throughout the cook time.

2. Strain the syrup through a fine mesh strainer and store in the refrigerator until ready to use.

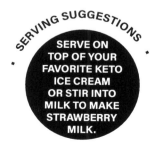

SERVING SUGGESTIONS

SERVE ON TOP OF YOUR FAVORITE KETO ICE CREAM OR STIR INTO MILK TO MAKE STRAWBERRY MILK.

YOU MAY ALSO LIKE

Please visit the below link for other books by the author

http://ketojane.com/books

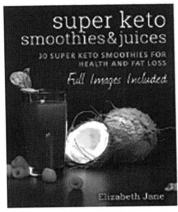
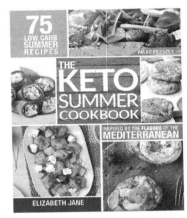
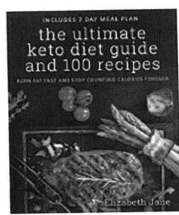
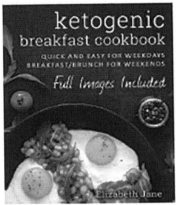
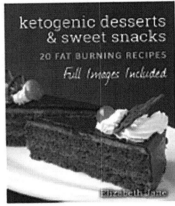
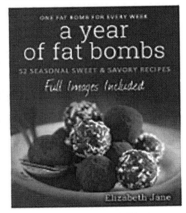
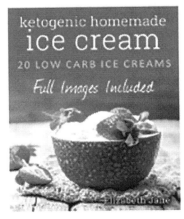
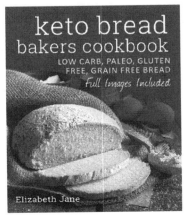
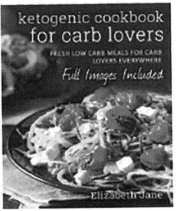

30056015R00059

Printed in Great Britain
by Amazon